THE
10-DAY
TOTAL
BODY
REVOLUTION

James Loomis

<ins>The 10-Day Total Body Revolution:</ins>

- ❖ A guide to encourage your renovation into superior health.

- ❖ The step-by-step process to undertake for the beginning of the rest of your life.

- ❖ Reveals truths that free your heart from past wounds.

- ❖ A mirror that shows the transformed person of your new future.

- ❖ Encouraging, uplifting and enlightening.

- ❖ Educates on the value of food choices and preparation techniques.

- ❖ Gives you confidence to pursue your life goals.

- ❖ Provides easy to follow lifestyle examples.

- ❖ Releases you from poor self-image.

- ❖ Illustrates practical guidelines how to purge toxins from your body.

- ❖ Goes beyond tradition to illustrate breakthrough techniques you can apply from day one for complete life changing, soul healing and mind transformation.

- ❖ Complete body rejuvenation methods from which you will be forever altered and able to live the life you always wanted to live.

This book is for informational purposes that are intended to be general advice on health care; it is not intended to be a substitute for medical advice of a licensed physician. The author is not a medical professional and nothing in this publication constitutes medical advice.

Any exercise program, including any exercise routines outlined in this publication, may result in injury. Any fitness program contains inherent risks of physical injury or death; always consult your physician prior to beginning any new exercise program to reduce the risk of injury. The information in this book is meant to supplement, not replace, proper training. The author advises readers to take full responsibility for their safety and know their limits.

This book is not intended as a substitute for doctor's advice, professional diagnosis, opinion, and treatment or services to you or to any other individual; it is presented AS IS. Always consult your doctor for your individual needs relating to your health, and regarding any symptoms that may require diagnosis or medical attention.

The author and publisher are not liable or responsible for any advice, course of treatment, diagnosis or any other information you obtain.

IF YOU BELIEVE YOU HAVE A MEDICAL EMERGENCY, YOU SHOULD IMMEDIATELY CALL 911 OR YOUR PHYSICIAN.

The 10-Day Total Body Revolution

ISBN 13:978-1726398497

ISBN 10:1726398498

Copyright 2018 by James and Janie Loomis

Atlanta, Texas 75551

Printed in the United States of America

Cover artwork and layout by Janie Loomis

Other Books by James and Janie Loomis

- ➢ Revolutionary Health

- ➢ 30 Days to a Healthy Spirit, Soul and Body

- ➢ Passionate Lover of God

- ➢ The Spirit of the Forerunner: A Cry Goes Out

- ➢ The Spirit of the Forerunner: The Legacy of One Who Has Gone Before

- ➢ The Spirit of the Forerunner: Mantles of Our Predecessors

- ➢ Empower the Forerunner Within You
    Study Guide

➢ Empower the Forerunner Within You
    Workbook and Journal

➢ Empower the Forerunner Within You
    Teachers Edition

For a growing list of on-line workshops and interactive courses you can take to further your *Revolution* in spirit, soul and body visit our website listed below.

Additional copies of this book or other books of the authors may be obtained via their website or Amazon and Amazon Kindle. You may also attend one of their conferences or seminars to pick up copies of books or Forerunner Merchandise. To schedule a speaking engagement, or contact the author, visit the website or send us a direct email:

www.forerunnerspirit.com

forerunnerspirit@gmail.com

Table of Contents

Dedication 7
Introduction: Join the Revolution 8
Chapter 1: To Drink and Not To Drink 12
Chapter 2: Forgiveness & Letting Go 17
Chapter 3: Exercise: Stretching,
          Aerobic, Anaerobic and HIIT 22
Chapter 4: Colorful Foods 28
Chapter 5: Meat, Eggs and Cheese:
          Protein Choices 37
Chapter 6: Fasting & Herbal Supplements 44
Chapter 7: Accountability=Friendship
          & Fellowship 51
Chapter 8: Taking Back What Was
          Stolen From You 55
Chapter 9: Your New Life:
          The Past IS the PAST 61
Chapter 10: Your New Mind:
          Being Positive-YES You Can 67
Chapter 11: Conclusion:
          Your New Daily Schedule 71
Selected Bibliography 77

DEDICATION

This book is dedicated to my wife
Janie Loomis.

Through her encouragement and belief in this project it could not have been completed. Through her diligence in researching foods, experimenting with innumerable combinations of herbs and spices and preparing incredible meals she has become an inspirational force the likes of which I have not witnessed heretofore.

Janie keeps me focused and centered on exercise routines, soul healing and is understanding when I take time away from us doing things together, so I may research medical conditions and compose newspaper columns and books.

My teenage sweetheart, whose infectious laughter, smile, quick wit, love and devotion are a prime stabilizing factor in my life.

I look forward to many more decades of marital bliss with my wife.

INTRODUCTION

Welcome to the Revolution! You are more than ready for a revolutionary change in how you feel, what you look like and how you think. With this determination and mind set, you set your mind like flint to the concept of change at any cost. Your health, your thought processes, your conceptualization of life itself will be altered during this Revolution; this is your moment, your time to become a completely new creature!

Revolutionary is defined as "involving or causing a complete or dramatic change". Additionally, it embodies the concepts "of pertaining to, characterized by, or of the nature of a revolution, or a sudden, complete or marked change". "Radically new or innovative, outside or beyond established procedure or principles", this is what you desire for the new you!

You are a revolutionist. Family, friends, co-workers, nearly everyone with whom you interact do not understand you nor do they want to associate with you due to your beliefs and practices. You want change. In yourself, in society, in church, in the marketplace, in relationships, in every level of society you see the need for change.

Our revolution is not *against* any political, social, religious, racial or relational strata of society. Our revolution *includes* every political party, every social status, every religion, and every race and ethnic group of people for their personal alteration into becoming a transformed person.

This revolution is of your mind, soul and body. It is a total transformational process. This quick guide will provide the basics for your transformation revolution.

Your mind must be rehabilitated to believe new practices, your soul must be healed of wounds and hurts to move forward, and your body must come into alignment with your mind (spirit) and soul. Soul wounds will be healed so that they no longer control what you eat and drink, what you believe about yourself and how you live your life.

Read the book. Take notes on what to do. Read the book again. Then change what needs to change. **DO WHAT YOU MUST DO FOR YOUR TRANSFORMATION**. You will see the beginning of your radicalized new life take shape in your mind, soul and body if you follow the instructions within this short manual.

You will lose weight and begin to tone up your muscles in 10 days if you follow the guidelines listed in this book. Of course, 10 days is just the introduction to this new way of thinking and living.

By enacting the precepts of *The 10-Day Total Body Revolution* over and over, enabling it to become your lifestyle you will see greater muscle strengthening and toning, achieve clarity of mind, healing of soul offenses and desire cleaner food and drink to consume rather than those that cause death and decay.

If you are under the care of a physician for an ailment and taking ANY type of medication you must be acutely aware of your body changes as you enact this program. Keep in contact with your medical provider. The taking of any pharmacological agent, whether prescription or off the shelf, causes extreme metabolic changes in your body.

Through this program, as you enact the precepts advocated, if you take ANY type of prescription drug or over the counter medicine, you will want and need those agents less and less. This is why it is important to inform your medical advisor how you are eating, the exercises you are doing and any organic supplements you are taking. EVERYTHING interacts with medication: exercise, lifestyle eating and drinking and especially your changed mind and heart.

Your body receives <u>*artificial*</u> agents such as flavors, sweeteners, multi-vitamins, pain relievers, gastro-intestinal medications and all types of laboratory-manufactured agents as foreign, toxic agents. A goal of your *Total Body Revolution* is to be completely free from any and all pharmaceuticals.

Herbal supplements and whole, natural, organic foods are recommended as a natural recourse compared to artificial treatments of any type. Herbal supplements will be covered extremely briefly in Chapter 6.

You MUST be proactive in your *Revolution*! You must take control over your cravings for harmful food and drink, laziness in exercise, stop making excuses, stop blaming ANYONE and get delivered from your addictions or contact me for deliverance and guidance.

This book is FULL of admonitions and guidelines. You are an adult and I treat you as such. I make lots of recommendations and suggestions on what to prepare and how to prepare various foods, but what you ultimately do is up to you. Make your own decisions on how you will *Revolutionize* your *Total*

Body, within the framework of these admonitions and suggestions.

This book is meant to be purposefully short and to the point. There is a tremendous amount of details that are left out so that this concise volume will be a quick read and an introduction to your new, altered lifestyle. It is short, so you will read it quickly, and then read it over and over and over again to remember what is being espoused then to "get on with your personal *Revolution*!" Research any topic more as you desire or contact me, I am here for you.

Only *you* can change you. Yes, we all need God's help and guidance. You have a brain and a free will to do whatever you want. Decide **TODAY** that NOTHING will stop you in your transformation, in your *Total Body Revolution* and in 10 days you will witness the beginning of your breakthrough into superior health for your spirit, soul and body.

Once you complete your *first 10-Day* transformative process, if you need a 1- or 2-day break that is okay, but then begin a second *10-Day Revolutionary* procedure. Your break is not to binge on bad food or stop working out or self-doubt; it can simply be a time of rest and self-reflection. Then get back on your new lifestyle and start another *10-Day Revolution*.

Join me now in the beginning of the regeneration of your mind, soul and body through *The 10-Day Total Body Revolution!*

CHAPTER 1

TO DRINK AND NOT TO DRINK

TO DRINK DAILY

Pure water, unsweet herbal tea, all natural smoothies or juices you make and Kombucha are your beverages of choice. These are the fluids your body can metabolise safely on a daily basis. You can safely drink up to ½ your body weight in ounces of water daily; some individuals may drink up to a gallon of water, according to many reliable medical sources. This amount of liquid includes unsweet herbal teas. Kombucha is an added nutritional "supplement" of which four to eight ounces daily is advisable.

Your kidneys need to be flushed of the toxins that accumulate and water is your best detoxifying agent. Depending on your current metamorphosing lifestyle, you probably have an immense amount of toxic agents floating around in your various body systems and organs that need to be flushed. Water and herbal teas are the best beginning rounds of detoxifying agents you can use.

If you currently or recently have taken any type of pharmacological agent, whether that is a prescription drug, over the counter or illegal drug, you need to flush these toxic agents from your system. You may need to go through specific medical addiction rehabilitation, depending on the severity of your symptoms of toxic shock or overload. Most of us just need to eat and drink right and our body will balance itself.

Alkaline water is the best. Get the finest water filtration system you can afford for your home and get your water tested. This is an investment you will want to make, due to the amount of water you will now be drinking. This purified water will be used for making your ice, teas, Kombucha and other fluid beverages.

Herbal teas are fantastic for their flavor and medicinal value. There are seemingly innumerable varieties. Try as many as you like, look for organic and without any sweetening agents or artificial ingredients. Steep for strength or weakness according to your taste, but do not add any sweeteners.

Smoothies and fresh juices you make are excellent on a daily or regular basis. These include almost any type and combination of vegetable, fruit and nut. Include almond or coconut milk, ice, spices and herbs, as you like. Try not to use any sweetening agent, however a little raw, local honey is acceptable.

When you make smoothies, begin with only whole, fresh fruit and vegetables. If you add ANY powders ONLY add 100% herbs or spices (such as cinnamon). No specialty "multi-vitamin" concoctions that cannot contain all the vitamins, minerals, and vegetables or fruit that are advertised. It is improbable and unreasonable to believe that you are "drinking" dozens of vegetables or fruits with a little scoop of some type of powder. These concoctions are often full of artificial flavors and sugars (read labels and research words you do not know). Do not use special protein liquids or any other "packaged" products. Use only real vegetables and fruit, no fake food. Your transformation is real and not found in **any** commercially manufactured powder or drink.

Kombucha is available in most grocery stores and health food stores. Look for it in the fresh vegetable sections of the stores or in specialty coolers. Try different varieties, only purchase unpasteurized and look for the "mother" floating on the bottom of the bottles. You can use these varieties to start making your own Kombucha and save yourself lots of money.

Homemade Kombucha is safe, inexpensive and you can make it according to your specific flavor tastes and preferences. Janie has been making our own Kombucha for some time and it is great to have a glass daily. The Internet is full of recipes on how to make your own Kombucha. Review them, gather your supplies and start today to make your own. You need Kombucha daily for your transformation.

TO DRINK SPARINGLY

Coffee, cider and caffeine drinks should be consumed sparingly.

The nutritional value of coffee is lost by the time you get the product to brew. It is just a drink full of caffeine that helps get or keep you going, but nutritionally is of no value. By the time we drink it, after being shipped from around the world, roasted in high heats and had who knows what ingredients added to the roasting or preservation process; coffee is a non-essential beverage that should only be consumed in moderation.

The strong coffees served at coffee houses with all the added sugars, spices and fats are extremely hazardous to our health and are contributing factors to obesity, diabetes, heart disease, joint pain and various types of cancers. Admit you are an addict, get delivered and set free from it's hold over you and either drop it completely or drink very little of this in the future.

TO DRINK NEVER

Alcohol (beer, wine and spirits), mixers for alcohol, sodas, sports drinks, energy drinks, energy shots, hard ciders and any other type of drink that is similar to these listed.

That is it; do not drink these drinks, ever again! Period! ***Exclamation Point!*** Get delivered, free from your addiction, and get over your hurt feelings. These all harm your body, have no nutritional value, lead to every disease known to the medical community and need to be a part of your past; not your present or your future.

It may not be easy to stop drinking these beverages, however if you want Crazy, Intense Exuberant Health you will stop consuming these immediately. Throw them out. Do not order them when you go out. Live a different lifestyle than you have previously. Yes, you can do it. Your body will feel much better and thank you for it.

CONCLUSION

In your total body revolution, begin with your choice of beverage. Thirst is only surpassed by our need for air; choose what quenches your thirst wisely.

CHAPTER 2

FORGIVENESS AND LETTING GO

In order to achieve your *Total Body Revolution*, you must forgive and let go of hurts and pains from your past. Forgiving those who have hurt us is often a process, like the peeling of an onion; one layer at a time-one hurt at a time. Time can be a factor in forgiveness but does not have to stretch out for decades. Let us walk through the process of forgiveness and letting go so you can achieve your *Total Body Revolution*.

There are innumerable books, articles and websites from many acclaimed individuals who have helped countless people to forgive and move forward in their life. I will be gleaning ideas from a few resources and will have them listed in the Bibliography for your further research.

<u>MOVE ON</u>

No matter who the people are or what they said or did in your past, you must forgive them and let them go.

Your past hurts, shame, regret and remorse must remain a part of your past; they are not a part of your present or future. Even if you still have to interact with some of these individuals, you purposefully do not allow them access to the parts of your innermost being as you did previously.

Realize they were a part of your life for a specific length of time, but not any longer. Do not allow thoughts to come up regarding them, or the past, as you let go of them their hold over you diminishes. You are creating a new reality without their influence everyday as you form new thoughts and beliefs.

If you are having difficulties in doing this, speak the following out loud:

"I release (insert their name) from hurting me. I forgive (insert their name) for everything he/she said and did to me. I will not allow the pain from my past to overwhelm me, keep me from moving forward or hold me back from my wonderful future. I am a free agent! I pronounce healing on my soul. I release my body from its bondage to past soul wounding and declare healing on my body. I am strong and able to do everything I was meant to do. I am a new being and look forward to a great future!"

If you just said that and feel like you still have pain or hurts from the past, read it again but this time louder and more forcefully. Decree your new position in life and be free from the past. Read it over and over as much as you need until you are free. I am telling you, you can be free, and this is a way in which to do so.

Now remember the past is in the past, leave it there and move on.

BLAME NO ONE

What has happened has happened. We must learn to move beyond blaming the other person(s) *and/or* blaming ourselves, to accepting what has happened and move on with our lives. The more we stay angry and resentful we seek blame and stay in a powerless mindset. In this position we become stagnant and putrefy.

Get to know yourself all over. Reinvent yourself. Become a new person. Blame no one, especially yourself. Your emotions can become fresh and alive, your mind is free from confusion and you get direction for the next step in your life's journey.

DO NOT TELL PEOPLE WHAT TO DO

Avoid the tendency to want to control people once you have come out of painful situations. Your determination to never allow "that" to ever happen to me or anyone else again sets you up to want to control and tell people what they should or should not do.

Allow others the grace to make their own decisions without a comment, eye roll or any type of utterance on your part. Their life is their life. If you want to help people, listen and pay attention to them, but do not give judgmental opinions. Comfort and reassure, help where and how you are able and permit them to live their life their way; not how you believe they should live.

TAKE PERSONAL RESPONSIBILITY

Become personally responsible for your life. No matter the circumstances, events, experiences, accidents, illness or victimization that you may have endured. When you take personal responsibility for your present and future you blame no one for your past and you move forward.

Learn from your experience. Understand how to avoid, if possible, what you had to undergo in the past and alter the life path you are on so as not to repeat the past. Own, without guilt, shame, fear or resentment your life experience and become responsible for your future by not reliving the past.

BECOME A GIVER

Give of yourself, your time, your energy, your emotions, your heart and soul. By giving of yourself you let go of yourself. There are many people in need: give a hug, a smile, a nod or an encouraging word. The more you give of yourself to those in need around you, the less you look at your own situation and hurts and focus outward instead of inward. Healing comes, as we look outward, not inward; then we are able to give of ourselves.

BE KIND AND NOT JUDGMENTAL

Learn how to treat others, as you would want to be treated. Be kind, respectful, and non-judgmental; look for goodness in people not hatred. The world is full of prejudice and fear, do not contribute to it but rather be a breath of fresh air.

Be an observer rather than a commentator. Bring peace, joy, love and hope to everyone with whom you encounter. Love and acceptance overcome all the pain and sorrow of the past and leads us to a bright tomorrow. Breaking the cycle of pain, judgment and resentment with pure love we set a new course for our lives and have a *Total Body Revolution*.

CONCLUSION

Forgiveness is a lifelong journey we walk out daily. As we are able to accept others, love the unlovable, keep silent and not always speak up, take personal responsibility for our lives, give of ourselves, blame no one and move on we position ourselves to become a transformed being. This new "creature" we become begins when our "insides" our soul and mind are revitalized. This altered being is then able to become transformed on the outside and realize a *Total Body Revolution*.

CHAPTER 3

EXERCISE: STRETCHING, AEROBIC, ANEROBIC & HIIT

Join a fitness center. Some centers are as inexpensive as $10.00 per month. Come on! You can afford $10.00; no more excuses! If you want to be a Revolutionary, you must revolutionize your body and the best way is through a fitness center. If you want a fitness trainer, utilize their expertise for your 10 days and extend the time if you so desire. Tell them what you are doing, how you want to improve and allow them to train you according to what you want. Push yourself. That is what this program is all about. Do what you have never done before, to achieve the results you have never been able to attain.

STRETCHING

Begin each day by getting up earlier than you need for your daily activities and stretch. Go outside to the back porch, watch the sun rise, make room in your living room or wherever you have space and begin a routine of stretching exercises.

Have you observed cats or dogs and how they act after a time of sleep? They get up and stretch. It is natural for them to do so. Follow their example.

Stretch all your muscle groups. Internet search for pictures of stretching exercises if you like. Stand erect loosening your limbs, gently shaking out your arms and then each leg. Turn your head to the right then left, forward and backwards holding for 2-3 seconds each. Repeat procedure while raising and lowering your shoulders.

Extend your arms out sideways, palms down and reach as far as you can, hold for 5 seconds. Keep arms out and turn palms upward, hold for 5 seconds. Slowly raise your arms, keeping elbows straight and reaching fully until arms are straight above your head, palms touching, and hold 5 seconds. Reach right arm out forwards and left backwards. Hold and twist so palms face opposite directions, all the while reaching as far as you can. Extend and retract fingers as you hold your arms out.

Remain in the same standing position, stretch out arms from sides for balance and begin to lift one leg at a time forwards then backwards, hold for 5 seconds. Stretch your legs as far as you can. Stand with your back straight against the wall and raise one leg at a time up until parallel with the ground.

Now let's do some back-stretching exercises. Lay on your back on the floor. Slowly raise one knee to your chest and hold for 5 to 10 seconds. Repeat using other leg. As you lay flat, twist your right leg over your left to be as perpendicular to your body as possible, hold then switch legs. Roll over onto your stomach, head up, elbows resting on floor beneath your head, pull your upper torso up so your palms are resting on the floor and you are arching your back, hold for 10 seconds. Get up to a sitting position, spread your legs, stretch your arms to hold your knees and slowly bend your head downward. Do not bend far, just enough so you can begin to feel a burn in your back.

Still in a sitting position, pull your legs back under your torso, stretch your arms forward over your head and bow your head to the floor. Hold for 5 to 10 seconds. Stay seated and raise your body back to a sitting position with arms raised up into the air over your head for 5 to 10 seconds. Repeat all procedures if you desire.

There are numerous types of stretching exercises you can do. Start with these, if you have other favorites do also those. The main objective is to spend at least 15 minutes daily stretching, if you can spend more time that is great; remember you are a revolutionary and everything is changing in your life!

AEROBIC EXERCISES

Types of aerobic exercises include, but not limited to spin bike, walking, swimming, jogging, treadmill walking, elliptical equipment, dancing, bicycle riding, cross country skiing, kickboxing and many others.

The type of "cardio" workout you are striving for is to get your heart beating faster. As you push yourself you feel yourself getting out of breath, your heart begins to pound, and you sweat!

Start out with at least 20 minutes then work your way up to at least 30 minutes daily. This is all about shocking your body into a radical transformation and to do so you must push yourself. As noted on the copyright page, if you are under the care of a physician for an illness or condition, consult with your doctor as you begin a new program.

If you have NEVER done anything like this previously, now is the time to start your Revolution! You will start losing weight as you exercise but will lose even more as your completely modify your eating and drinking habits.

<u>ANEROBIC EXERCISES</u>

Weight training is essential to your reformation. Talk to your trainer or someone at the gym about what you want and need toned. You need strong knees so work your leg muscles to strengthen your stance. You lose weight through overall working out (and especially through your changed eating and drinking habits), but increase your core strengthening to lose the fat around your belly, hips and thighs.

Work your arms and shoulders. Women and men need muscle definition and upper body strength. You need the strength and stamina to carry loads and go about your daily activities. Regardless what you do you must strengthen your body!

Ask questions at the center about the different weight training machines and free weights. For the first 2 days, push, but get comfortable with the workout; then kick it up for the next 8 days. You should be on the weights for at least 30 minutes daily; increase to 45-60 minutes as you can. Yes, this is your new life. You work out; you MAKE the time in your schedule to be healthy. This is the NEW you.

Do not give up. You are in a Revolution. This is your *Total Body Revolution*. This Revolution is accomplished through this aspect of exercise. Yes, every chapter in this book is key to your success, yet you have got to exercise if you want to see results.

HIIT

High-Intensity Interval Training is a type of workout that alternates between intense bursts of activity and fixed periods of less intense activity. These types of workouts can be done in or out of the fitness center.

Examples of HIIT are biking as fast as you can for 2 minutes then going slow for 5 minutes. Running as fast as you can for 30 seconds then walking for 5 minutes. Push yourself hard on the elliptical machine for 2 minutes then go slow for 10 minutes. There are endless variations of this type of training and the benefits are astronomical! You can utilize this style of workout with any exercise routine. Use this method every other day allowing your body to recover in-between if you are really pushing yourself.

HIIT is great for cardio vascular training, fat burning and strengthening your heart. You can use equipment but it is not necessary. As you increase your metabolism to do these routines more often and longer, you can do this training anywhere and anytime and it is extremely challenging if you push yourself.

There are any numbers of exercises you can do: running, sprints, jumping, swimming, and running in place, lifting, crunches, oblique crunches, stationary bike, regular bike riding, push-ups, jumping jacks, burpee, jump rope, planking, high knee lifts, squat jumps, lunges, stair stepper, battle rope and so much more.

CONCLUSION

Gear up to work out! Your Revolution consists of exercise, altered food and drink choices, soul healing and thinking modification. Every aspect is co-dependent upon the other and a *Total Body Revolution* cannot be attained without each factor transfigured.

Work out, work out hard, sweat and begin to feel your muscles ache. As you incorporate every aspect of your *Revolution*, you begin to feel changes throughout your body, soul and mind. You can do it! You must do it to be the *Revolutionary* that **everyone** around you needs you to become. Develop into the example setter of your revolutionary new lifestyle. Be the leader that you are and were created to be. Get ready for your new you!

CHAPTER 4

COLORFUL FOODS

The types of foods you eat, their color, texture, and manufactured status revolutionize your body. One way or the other, good or bad, they alter your physique. It is time to take back your strength and vitality through the way you think about foods, how you prepare them and what you actually consume.

I cannot possibly detail every individual food you should eat; yet I will provide groupings, so you understand my ideas. Spend time in the fresh produce section of your grocery store and local farmers markets; and search the Internet for the nutritional benefits of every type of produce, seed, bean and nut.

FOODS TO EAT

You must *learn to like* colorful foods. Examples of the food types you now consume are: blue, green, yellow, orange and red.

Foods that have life, energy, complex carbohydrates and proteins; these are your new staples. Think vegetables, dried beans and peas, fruits, nuts, seeds and grains. The more wholesome foods you consume the more your allergies, asthma, skin disorders and other conditions will slowly diminish; believe me, I have seen this happen in many people. Your bodily strength will increase, weight decrease, and transformation will happen to your eating habits.

Greens include cruciferous vegetables (broccoli, Brussel Sprouts and cabbage) a huge variety of leafy greens (spinach, kale, chard, watercress and innumerable lettuces) apples, avocado and many more. Take your time in the produce section. Purchase all types of green vegetables and fruit, _the whole actual fruit or vegetable_. An apple and an avocado a day keeps the doctor away! Remember this saying, eat them and get healthy.

Orange/yellow types include sweet potatoes, carrots, winter squash, nectarines, apricots, peppers and more. Have a carrot (a whole, full sized carrot) every day for the beta-carotene for your eyes and cholesterol lowering properties for your heart. Sweet potatoes, with only light good fat and no sweeteners are a fantastic food. Do an Internet search right now on all the benefits of sweet potatoes. Have 1-2 per week.

Red foods include apples, raspberries, cranberries, radishes, strawberries, cherries, plums, rhubarb, watermelon, onions, peppers, beets, cabbage, leafy vegetables and more. Every day choose these foods for extreme nutrition and health. You <u>MUST</u> learn to eat beets; look up the health nutrients in them right now, your taste buds can and will change so you can enjoy them regularly.

Berries and grapes are blue, black and red and are utterly unbelievable when picked fresh. They retain their nutritional value when frozen. Pick and eat fresh when they come in seasonally then freeze back extra for smoothies and to include in oatmeal.

<u>FATS</u>

The good fats you will now use are avocado, olive and coconut. There are a few others that are healthy, but for your *Revolution* and revitalization avoid EVERY OTHER KIND OF FAT except these three.

Use these three approved fats sparingly. I use a teaspoon of coconut oil in my morning coffee. No more than 2 teaspoons daily. Oils for sautéing vegetables are acceptable, yet in extremely small quantities; learn to use water in your good cooking pots and pans instead of fats. Your brain and body need fat, but only the right type and quantity.

The bad fats are EVERY other type of oil, grease and lard that is out there. If you have ANY other type of oil product in your home (besides the 3 approved ones) throw them out IMMEDIATELY! Any other fat is unacceptable for your *Total Body Revolution*.

You no longer eat greasy fried foods and extremely limit yourself or have eliminated crackers, chips, cookies, cakes, pies and other snack pastries from your lifestyle, so you are not consuming bad fats. If you still consume these "foods" you must IMMEDIATELY (yes, there is that word again) reduce to eradicate them from your life.

Remember you are a *Revolutionary*, you do not willingly submit yourself to a food death sentence and you do not allow your body cravings or addictions to rule your life anymore. You overcome your addictions to be free to be all you are meant to be.

FOODS NOT TO EAT

Essentially you want to decrease, avoid or eliminate animal meat and white "foods". Animal meat leads to many types of cancers, heart disease, obesity, diabetes, high blood pressure, high cholesterol, stroke and many other conditions. Most people are addicted to animal meat and think they need it to live; this is a completely wrong belief.

Only 2 ounces of protein is needed daily for the nourishment of a 160-pound person. Research this for yourself with the CDC and the National Institutes of Health. If you eat more than what your body needs, and you do not utilize strenuous exercise for muscle building your body stores the excess energy as fat. More chicken is consumed than ever before and more Americans are fatter than ever before-think about it!

You need to build muscle. You need to work out. You need protein. If you consume animal protein, make it as lean as possible and as little as possible. Include more plant protein and less animal protein in your regime.

Your body can get all the protein it needs from plants. Beans/peas (there is a gigantic variety from which to choose), nuts seeds and grains (quinoa, kamut, teff, coucous, flax, chia, hemp, millet, spelt, amaranth, buckwheat and rye) are a few examples of plant based protein sources (research for yourself).

White foods include white flour, breads, pasta, rice, crackers, cereals and sugar. Look in your pantry, refrigerator and freezer; discard what is unhealthy. You are a *Revolutionary*! Act like a *Revolutionary*! Believe it and take your stand.

HOW TO PREPARE YOUR FOOD

Eat raw vegetables and fruit throughout the day, sauté vegetables, and use a crock-pot to cook beans/peas and to make stews and soups. Write me for food preparation ideas, recipes, or for fresh ideas/concepts.

Vegetables, beans/peas and seeds should be ¾ of your daily food consumption. Fruit is great but loaded with natural sugar. If you are diabetic or have specific health conditions where you need to be careful about sugar, do Internet searches on the sugar content of your favorite fruits and adjust consumption accordingly.

Cooking dried beans or peas is easy; Janie and I have been doing so for years. Get away from canned ANYTHING, especially beans. Choose a type of bean you want to prepare, say Cranberry Beans (one of our personal favorites). Soak the beans in a bowl overnight with some baking soda (to help reduce gas). For every cup of beans/peas soaked, use a tablespoon of baking soda.

The next morning rinse the beans in a colander while running your fingers through them, being sure to get out all the baking soda and any "skin" of the beans that may peel away. Get out your crock-pot and put 2 cups of water for every 1 cup of beans you cook. Cook on low heat all day, they will be fine. Season, as you like with minimal to no salt. We love garlic, oregano, dill, rosemary, cumin, turmeric and many other spices, try different seasonings and spices with every batch.

Additives to your beans are as you desire. Leave them plain to discover their flavor at first then add any vegetable you like. Make a soup or stew out of the crock-pot. Salsas, chilies, nuts, seeds or whatever you want; these are your concoctions so have fun and experiment in the kitchen.

Cook the beans plain more often and prepare them once cooked as pastes, dips and as the main ingredient in your "vegie-burgers". We have black bean burgers all the time and love them. Combine the cooked beans with a cooked grain to give them texture and season to taste.

Experiment with herbs and spices. There are a plethora of types, flavors and heat levels. Try new types every week. Include them in your meal prep and on the table. Lose the saltshakers. If you still use salt use only extremely sparingly and do not leave shakers on the table or by the stove.

IN REVIEW

Eat your vegetables!

Eat more dried beans and peas. Eat more seeds and REAL whole grains. Eat less often as you move to abolish pre-processed, prepared meals from your lifestyle.

Do not be stressed about cooking this way. Do not get lazy and say you do not have time. Remember, you are a *Revolutionary* and do not do what "everyone" else is doing; "everyone else" is fat and sick and tired all the time. You do not want to *be* like "everyone else" so you *do not do* what "everyone else" is doing!

Visit all kinds of grocery stores, health food stores, and farmers markets or anywhere that sells fresh produce. Experiment with taste, texture and "new to you" foods. Talk to chefs; produce managers and farmers on how they prepare vegetable dishes and then make the time to prepare your own creations.

This is your new life. The old has passed away, you are a new person and you will not go back to your old, unhealthy habits. You want, NO you NEED deep within you that altered/transformed life and nothing will keep you captive to disease, pain and death that was foretold you by the medical community or family or friends.

YOU are ***REVOLUTIONIZING*** your life and your resolve will keep you focused on your new, great future that is within your grasp. Hold tight. Do not let go. Stay the course and you will succeed.

CONCLUSION

Eat colorful foods and reduce to do away with: meat, bad fats, eggs, dairy products, and sugar and white food products from your extraordinary new life! Millions of people have already done this; I am right there with you in this *Revolution*. I am not a purist, but a realist. I have not completely attained the level I desire, but am working it daily through determination, steadfast heartfelt, realistic passion that will not be diminished nor discouraged.

I push myself onward even when others distract me or try to swerve me off course. I know who I am and what I want for my future. I have clearly defined goals for my life in 10 days, 10 years and beyond. Get this for yourself. Set short term and long-term goals, such as one new vegetable or dried bean type a month. Set mid-term goals such as, two seasons from now I will have lost 15 pounds or 4 inches. This mid-term goal could also be to add muscle mass to be able to easily carry a 50-pound bag of beans.

Long term goals for years in the future could entail being completely drug free, disease and illness free (the CDC states that chronic diseases can be cured), do various physical activities you currently are unable to do, vacation somewhere new and exciting, wear the dress size or pants size you always wanted, be able to run with your children or grandchildren without being exhausted; the list is endless. Set lofty goals and then work hard, work HARD to attain them and you will succeed!

Do not beat yourself up if you are not 100% "there" at the end of your first *10-Days*; do the best you can but take big steps in the right direction. You can do it. If you need encouragement contact me via our website. Let's work together in the *Revolution*.

CHAPTER 5

MEAT, EGGS & CHEESE: PROTEIN CHOICES

I mentioned in the previous chapter our need to decrease our consumption of or remove meat, eggs and dairy (especially cheese) from our lifestyle; I will develop and expand on that concept here. Too many people this is a foreign and abhorrent idea while to others it is a normal way of life. We must move away from tradition, culture, habit and laziness to form a NEW tradition, NEW culture and NEW habit that do not revolve around any type of destructive behaviors.

MEAT

Animal protein is beef, chicken, pork and all wild game. I also include fish and shellfish. If it is a living creature, do not kill it so you can eat it. It is that simple. I believe humans were created not to need to eat the flesh of other living creatures for their own sustenance. To me it is the epitome of arrogance, self-aggrandizement, abuse and so, so much more.

I admit I was raised eating meat and occasionally succumb to my baser instinct and give in to my addiction. Since 2013 my wife and I have been consuming less and less meat/fish products as we inform ourselves of the toxins, artificial hormones and trauma that the creatures we consumed were subject to in their lives. What we eat, we absorb into our spirit, soul and body. If we eat traumatized creatures that were injected with all types of drugs we willingly ingest their trauma and toxins thereby contaminating our entire being and become sick in our spirit, soul and body.

It has been only since January 2018 that we have purposefully and specifically tried to refrain from eating any formally living creature. There have been times when we have eaten small quantities of animal products, but these times are less and less with each month that passes.

Our oceans have been and continue to be increasingly contaminated with innumerable toxic chemicals and trash so that living creatures are dying off at a rapid pace. Those remaining are being infected with heavy chemicals like mercury so their meat is unhealthy. "Factory farmed" shrimp and tilapia along with other creatures are tainted with bacterial agents and chemicals so that their toxicity levels are astronomical!

My wife and I owned a deli and gourmet health foods manufacturing company. During this time I attended many safe food preparation and handling courses. The number of pathogens, worms, bacteria and fungi that inhabit shellfish enlightened me to new levels of awareness of their extreme dangers.

Besides my admonition to avoid these "foods" for your *Total Body Revolution*, no person should eat any type of shellfish due to of their extremely deadly nature.

Shellfish include: shrimp, clams, scallops, muscles, oysters, abalone, octopus, squid, lobster, crab and crayfish. Under ***no*** circumstance should you eat ***ANY*** of these creatures. If you eat them your body will become contaminated and you consent to receive innumerable diseases and illnesses.

Hear me clearly-it is by your own doing, if you eat ***ANY*** of these creatures and develop an illness or condition because of the inherent dangers, pathogens, bacteria, fungi and artificial hormones and chemicals that reside in these previously living beings. Now you know the truth and are responsible for it. The leading causes of death can be traced to the harmful foods and drinks we consume.

Remember, you are in a revolution. Your thought processes are changing. Your lifestyle activities are changing. Your eating and drinking habits are changing. _**IF**_ you do not change, you will become sick and diseased easier and younger than those who do revolutionize their life. You cannot continue to maintain the old lifestyle and be a revolutionary. _**IF**_ you are a revolutionary, you will begin to alter your lifestyle eating habits and you **will** become healthy.

<u>EGGS</u>

Eggs from any creature are not healthy to eat. Eggs are the embryo of unborn birds, reptiles, mammals and fish. Consider what you put into your body, the unborn embryo of a bird or fish?

The yoke of the egg is full of cholesterol, which is inflammatory to your body. This inflammation leads to heart disease, high cholesterol, various cancers, stroke and many other illnesses. By willingly consuming eggs you allow yourself to become weak, sick and live a shortened lifespan due to the illnesses they cause.

I used to eat up to a dozen eggs a week. My total cholesterol and triglycerides were through the roof. Overnight in January 2018 I drastically decreased my consumption of eggs. I did not have any withdrawal symptoms or problems. In the first half of 2018, I have eaten out twice at a "breakfast" restaurant ordering an egg meal and had French toast on two other occasions; that is all the eggs I ate.

Since my decrease to cessation of eating eggs, my total blood cholesterol count has greatly reduced, and my triglycerides levels have come down to the healthy range. It did not take long. By my "combination therapy" of no eggs, extreme reduction to elimination of meat and increased exercise, I am much healthier.

Further educate yourself to the dangers of eggs.

CHEESE AND DAIRY PRODUCTS

Americans are addicted to cheese. Casein is a protein found in milk that when being digested releases opiates called casomorphins. Researchers believe casomorphins are released into the bloodstream to ensure that babies desire to continue to nurse during infancy to help survive. Each time we consume **ANY** type of dairy product we are drugging ourselves.

The quantity of this drug is minimal, yet enough to cause us to be addicted to dairy products. Milk, cheese, yogurt, sour cream, ice cream, cream cheese and the list goes on with the countless variants of each product. This helps explain the overweight/obesity epidemic facing the United States.

You can end your addiction. You can be free from the intoxication and cravings you have for dairy products. Anytime you MUST have a certain food product, you are under its control and you submit yourself to its consequences.

Baby cows need the milk of their mother cow; baby or adult humans do not need the milk of a cow. Only humans drink the mammary secretions of another mammal. Think about it; wake up from your slumber. Baby elephants do not drink the milk of cows, nor do baby cows drink the milk of a horse. Common sense dictates that humans should not drink the milk of cows, nor any products derived from cow's milk.

Please use common sense when eating and drinking. Break your addiction to dairy products and start living drug free. We must awaken from our slumber. Think what you are eating and drinking before you mindlessly eat products that are not normal for you to ingest. You are not a cow you are a human being!

Do your own research. Look up the danger of dairy products. Read the reports, listen to the doctors illustrate the facts, use reason and break free from your addiction. We need to WAKE UP, become free from our addictions and do not look back. There is real freedom when we break free of our bondages and realize newfound strength and health simply by letting go of what once held us captive.

CONCLUSION

Animal meat, eggs and cow dairy products are not necessary for your nourishment, survival or strength. Tradition, culture, comfort-food-addiction, advertising and availability in restaurants lend us to give in to foods that harm rather than heal our bodies.

To be a *Revolutionary*, you MUST do revolutionary acts. Eating and drinking like everyone else is being a follower, not a leader. If you want to be an agent of change to those with whom you associate, if you want to live an extra-ordinary life; if you want to be stronger, healthier and happier than ever before-you WILL do revolutionary acts.

Join the revolution; you can do this <u>AT LEAST</u> for 10 days.

After the **first** ten days of your personal Revolution, you will see how you altered your lifestyle. You will begin to feel a difference in your body. You will realize that you do not want to go back to the *old* you. Times are changing. You are changing. There is only death behind you. Go forward into your new life!

Break your addiction to these death foods by immediately discarding ANY you have in your home. Research alternate foods and contact me for additional information on this subject. Look at vegan ideas on the Internet and reread this book over and over and over again to get the concepts espoused here deep into your brain, heart and soul. You can change; millions of people already have and are living extremely healthy and happy lives.

Join the *Revolution*. Become a *Revolutionary*. Alter yourself and you alter your world!

CHAPTER 6

INTERMITTENT FASTING & HERBAL SUPPLEMENTS

The benefits of fasting and 100% organic herbal and/or spice supplements are simply outrageous!

Fasting may be specific to a type of food or drink, a period of time or particular activity; you can personalize your fast to your particular wants, needs or desires. The results of your fast will be based upon from what you fast and the duration of your fast.

For a *Total Body Revolution*, you need to consider what type of fast(s) you will undertake, its duration and most importantly, the specific reason for your fast.

Herbal supplements should be a staple in your life. These should be 100% individual organic herbs and spices. For your *Revolution* you will **_not,_** let me repeat that, **_YOU WILL NOT_** use any type of multi-vitamin, pre-packaged, mass produced container of innumerable ingredients. You WILL discard ANY and ALL these types of products from your home. For the most part, these types of products are unsafe, created who knows where in the world, under questionable manufacturing practices and of dubious intrinsic nutritional value, regardless of the hype, testimonials or "celebrities" who indorse them-do not take them!

Pure individual, specific herbs and spices are what you need and should take. We will illustrate a few for reference purposes. Your job is to research on your own your medical condition, if any, and investigate if there are specific herbs and spices that will help your condition. Plants have amazing healing qualities and should be regularly consumed for natural healing. I take an average of 20,000 milligrams of 100% organic, herbal supplements daily and I am in GREAT physical condition!

INTERMITTENT FASTING

Fasting is normally the abstention of all food and drink for a specific period of time. The human body needs fluids to survive second only to oxygen. If you desire to undertake a complete fast, you may need to have medical supervision. Complete fasts are the best, however refraining from food while drinking water is great.

If you are exercising daily, as previously recommended, you may not be able to fast for more than a meal period or two. Use common sense when fasting and exercising. When I work out early in the mornings I can usually fast food until lunchtime, (I do not fast daily) but by then I get light headed if I do not eat. On days when I do not work out extensively, I know I can fast the entire day.

The longer you are able to fast from foods the greater the benefits you will attain, until you get to the point of physical exhaustion and depletion. Remember your goal is to cleanse your body of toxins, not harm it.

Fasting benefits include: improving insulin sensitivity, enhancing cognitive effects and neuroprotection, increased longevity and health, purging of cancerous and precancerous cells, decrease in fat tissue, a rapid shift into nutritional ketosis and decrease in oxidative stress and inflammation throughout your body.

Additional benefits of fasting include: cellular detoxification, reduction of belly fat, enhanced brain functioning, reduction in Alzheimer's risk, better sleep, clearer skin, increased concentration, relaxation of metabolic body processing systems, tissue repair, increased immunity, and increased stability of moods, enhanced liver functioning and a reduction in allergic reactions.

Consider the type of fast you want to undertake, the results you want to experience, the length of time of the fast and the regular lifestyle tasks you will assume during your fast.

Examples of fasts you can do during your *10-Day Total Body Revolution* include: fasting from all meat, eggs and dairy, fast any food consumption after dinner until lunch the next day, fast from ALL sweet drinks, fast food during daylight hours but consume liquids, fast food you chew but consume homemade vegetable smoothies for the day. The type and variety of your fasts are up to you. When you do fast you assist your body in its repair functions and you grow continuously healthier.

HERBAL SUPPLEMENTS

Think about the supplements you take. If you take a multi-vitamin, consider how the manufacturer was able to put 100% of the vitamins and minerals in that little tablet. From where are the ingredients sourced? What type of manufacturing process was utilized to get all those ingredients into that pill? Do you abhor processed foods and pre-packaged meals, but take multi-vitamins? Are you being "double minded" or inconsistent in your beliefs and practices?

Think beyond the hype, the nutritional promises, testimonials and professional promoters of the type of supplement you take. Look again at the ingredients list, research how and where the product was manufactured and double think the price you are paying. Research the names and types of sugar and artificial sugars that may be in your product. I will tell you from first-hand experience, I was in the herbal supplement manufacturing business; the raw ingredients are not expensive.

The following extremely selective list of herbal supplements has many benefits, is easy to find, are relatively inexpensive, and are extremely efficacious. Do your own research to your medical condition(s) and start taking herbal supplements.

Garlic. First thing in the morning cut up 1-2 cloves of garlic, put a little local, raw honey on your spoonful of garlic and swallow. Calms inflammation, fight viral and bacterial infections, lowers cholesterol, blood pressure and blood glucose levels. Everyone needs more garlic. I have done this daily for years.

Olive Leaf Extract. Take at least 2,000 mg daily. Regulates blood glucose levels (fights diabetes), antioxidant, anti-inflammatory, lowers blood pressure and cholesterol has many other benefits and helps reduce belly fat. A friend, due to Janie's insistence, started taking Olive Leaf Extract and she gradually reduced her dependency on insulin and other diabetes drugs. She is much better and takes very little insulin today.

St. John's Wort. I take 2,000 mg daily. I had nerve damage in my left leg after a back surgery; the doctor said I would end up in a wheelchair. I started taking St. John's Wort, have regained feeling in my left leg (it was constantly numb) and can run like crazy. It relieves nerve pain and brings dead nerves back to life. I am a living testimony to St. John's Wort; it definitely works!

Pau d' Arco. Scientifically proven with numerous testimonials from around the world how it kills cancerous tumors. My wife had a nodule growing on her thyroid gland. Doctors wanted to radiate and/or cut out her thyroid gland. Janie said no to the medical procedures and started taking a minimum of 3,000 mg of Pau d' Arco daily. Her thyroid functions properly today without surgery or radiation due to this herb. Again, personal testimony to how it really is effective.

Turmeric, Ginger and Cinnamon. Use daily in water, tea, coffee, sprinkle on foods, take as a supplement; any way you can. Anti-inflammatory, improves digestion, reduces heart disease, and fights infections, antioxidant, and boosts immunities, antibacterial, antiviral and so much more. Everyday use these powerful healing spices.

Fenugreek, Wild Yam Root and Black Cohosh. For menopause and monthly menstrual cycles, these herbs are calming, soothing and healing that assist the woman's body during these times. You may safely take 1,000 mg of each of these herbs daily.

<u>CONCLUSION</u>

Ramp up your nutrition, healing, strength and vitality by fasting and taking all natural, 100% organic herbal supplements on a regular basis. Research specific diseases you want to protect yourself against and start taking those specific supplements.

Fasting is extremely beneficial, yet if exercising intensely use with caution. A good way to begin is no food after dinner (eat early) and then do not eat until lunch the next day. Allow your body to rest from metabolizing constantly from a continual influx of food.

CHAPTER 7

ACCOUNTABILITY

=

FRIENDSHIP & FELLOWSHIP

Buddy up! Increase your friends on Facebook, followers on Instagram and any other social media site to which you belong.

Talk to strangers at the grocery store, church, work, and the restaurants you frequent.

Reach out and put yourself out there. Sure, people will not like you for whatever crazy reason they come up with, but that is okay. You keep being friendly.

Someone once said to a group of people, "If you want a friend, be a friend."

No one is an island we need each other. To achieve your *Total Body Revolution*, you need to interact with people, have a confidant, a person who you can share your victories and failures. Someone that can be real to you and you can reciprocate. If you do not have such a compatriot, reach out to people and develop friendships. You have to trust people, give of yourself, be willing to get emotionally hurt; but to also grow stronger in your soul, realize you need human interaction and you will learn real love.

DEVELOPING ACCOUNTABILITY

Be a leader, a role model. Be confident in your speech and actions. Do not be overbearing, controlling or domineering, but be realistic and accessible. As a leader, lead the people around you by your example. You do not do what everyone else does, not to be different for difference sake, but because you naturally see life events and circumstances differently.

Communicate your vision. Inform people of your beliefs, how you believe what you do and how your actions follow up your speech. Be tactful and straightforward, you will not develop friendships if you moan and groan or whine and carry on to everyone, no one likes a "whiner" or a "grump". Be positive in your communications. Be open and accessible.

Reach out and be vulnerable. Join new groups on social media. When you are at the fitness center talk to people and be friendly. Join a book club, a stretch class, or a walking club at work; better yet start any of these or other types of "clubs". Be realistic and talk to people similar in thoughts and beliefs but reach out to those who look completely different than you. Do not be afraid of people of a different race than you; we are all people-brothers and sisters-get comfortable talking to everyone.

Being alone is not an option. In your *Total Body Revolution* you **MUST** become accountable and accessible to people. Individuals who join weight loss groups where everyone weighs in together and share success stories are much more successful than the online groups where everyone maintains their anonymity.

Partner up. Ask someone if you can be accountable to her or him. Ask them to help you in your weight loss, strength training, and meal preparation ideas. Get together with your accountability partner at least once per week. Encourage each other, share successes and failures, go jogging, biking or work out together. Share a healthy meal and be accountable, realistic and goal setting with each other. You need that person in your life just as much as that person needs you.

DO NOT GO IT ALONE!

CONCLUSION

None of us were meant to be alone. We are social creatures and need each other. "They" need you just as much as you need them.

Join a church, get involved in a small group within that church and develop friendships and people with whom you can be accountable.

Join a weight loss accountability group; there are many different types. Ask the people who run your fitness center, what kinds of classes they offer and get involved.

Be the leader you are and start SOME TYPE of group at work or in your neighborhood. Reach out and be vulnerable and ask people to join your group. Develop camaraderie with your peers and learn how to help those that need help

Go to a high school sporting event even if you could care less about any type of sports! Socialize with people around you at the event and get excited with everyone. Get out there and get involved.

To have a *Total Body Revolution* you must interact with people. This is so you are accountable, vulnerable and can start to heal any wounds you have in your soul. This concept will be covered in our next chapter. As you are healed on the inside you are able to develop good relationships and get the final breakthrough you need for every aspect of your life.

The *Total Body Revolution* is more than just having a great looking body, it is a strong and secure soul, a life free from any addiction and being able to interact fully and completely with people as the leader you were created to be.

CHAPTER 8

TAKING BACK WHAT WAS STOLEN FROM YOU

This chapter is about inner healing. We need to be healed on the inside, so we can project that healing on the outside. As we strengthen our inner person, our soul, as we become healed from any soul wounds we can move forward in our lives in a more productive and positive way.

Reread chapter two. Read it at least twice before going on in this chapter.

This is not some weird esoteric concept, but it has real life value. To completely receive your *Total Body Revolution* you need to think about some perhaps difficult concepts, work through and overcome them. In so doing you free yourself to live in a new freedom that you may never have previously walked.

<u>GET FREE</u>

Family, friends, jobs, co-workers, employers, neighbors, teachers, spouses, children, parents, administrators, pastors, political leaders, law enforcement officers and a myriad of others may have hurt you in the past. They could have stolen something from you that may never be recovered. Because of their actions, perhaps you are at a loss (physically, emotionally, financially or other ways); hurt, perhaps angry, bitter, afraid, sorrowful, lonely, empty or distressed beyond seeming reconciliation.

It is time to take back what was taken from you! It is time to achieve a level of freedom you may not have experienced ever or in a long, long time. For your *Total Body Revolution* you must be free from past harmful associations, ties and/or bondages. This is accomplished in many ways, a few of which we will go over here.

Start with chapter 2 of this book. Forgive the unforgivable. Move on, let go, blame no one, take personal responsibility for your life as it now is and become a giver, be kind and non-judgmental. These are the first steps. Give more than you receive.

Read the following out loud so your ears can hear your words and they reside within the atmosphere around you:

"I forgive those who have hurt me. I release my past hurts, disappointments and failures. I release my abusers and false accusers from my heart and soul. I will not allow them to control my thoughts, life, actions, reactions, friendships, job or any aspect of my life anymore!" Repeat this as often as you need and get louder and more forceful every time you repeat it.

Through your declarations you speak life into your heart and soul. If there are specific people you need to name, name them. Speak their names out and release their control over your life. If there are specific incidents or instances that you cannot seem to overcome, speak them out and say I let go of their control over my life.

Declare you are free from the bondage of self-doubt; declare it out loud. Declare out loud you are free from pain and sorrow, free from grief and regret, free from loved ones who are deceased whom although you love seem to hold you back from moving forward. Declare these concepts and people out loud. Declare them now, right now as you are reading this. Put the book down and make these declarations. Let them all go.

GET FREE!

TAKE BACK

Now, take back your life. The action of decreeing out loud is a major step in achieving freedom in your life. Once you are unshackled from anything and/or everything that has held you back you are free to take back what was stolen from you.

Now it is time to decree your new life into existence. As you did in your declaration, now speak out loud your decrees:

"I decree life, happiness, freedom, peace and love to be a part of my life. I decree release from all past hurt, shame, loneliness, abuse, sorrow, fear, pain, suffering, failures, regret and soul-bondages. I decree all persons in positions of authority over my life in the past are released from all power and influence over me now and forever!

"I decree a freedom to love. I decree a new power to walk and talk as never before. I decree my eyes to be open to see life from a new perspective and my ears to hear words of encouragement. I decree a new hope to direct my life that I may have never experienced before."

Now, make any further decrees you need to make. As before, name names, incidents and life virtues that you desire to have in your life. Pronounce over yourself: companionship, peace and optimism and any other concept that you believe needs to flow through your life. Attain these freedoms and virtues for yourself, and then you will be able to share them with everyone you encounter.

You are a leader. You are a *Revolutionary*. You must bring *Revolutionary* concepts to hurting people.

BE FILLED

Now it is time to open your heart and soul and receive healing through your verbal announcements. Speak out loud to your heart and soul and say, "Be filled with peace, rest, hope and contentment.'

Continue speaking out-loud saying: "I am full of love and able to love. I am able to give love and hope to everyone. I look forward to today and tomorrow, because I am free to be everything I was created to be. I am a new person today! I am full of love, grace, mercy and kindness."

Walk now in your new freedom and exude love and contentment as a *Revolutionary*.

<u>CONCLUSION</u>

Feel free to make your verbal declarations, decrees and announcements out loud as often as you want. In your new freedom you can free others that are in bondage. *Total Body Revolution* is more than you getting stronger and eating and drinking differently. It is becoming an agent of change, a *Revolutionary* to those who need to be reinvigorated and set free from any and all hindrances in their life.

As you were making your decrees and declarations you were probably extremely emotional. That is good. Cry and let go everything and anything that has held you back; be it a few days ago or many decades. The release of tears is a sign of change. You need that change on the inside so that you can change on the outside. Inner healing is necessary prior to any type of outer change.

If you feel you have become "cleansed" of your inner hurts, fantastic! Daily a barrage of events comes against us that can cause us to revert to self-doubt, self-accusation and a myriad of other emotions. As you feel the desire, reread this chapter and make your own decrees and declarations over your life and situations.

As you feel heaviness from worldly events, stress and pressures revisit your inner self and become healed of anything that holds you back. Do this so you may move forward.

Be the leader, the agent of change, the *Revolutionary* that your world needs. Take up the challenge.

CHAPTER 9

YOUR NEW LIFE: THE PAST *IS* THE PAST

Fat, diseases, poor eating habits, "friends" that use you, family that hurts you, poor self-esteem; the list is endless of what you want to leave in your past. More than hurts and disappointments that have no place in your future, there are countless traits that you need to let go of and other, positive, new healthy lifestyle habits you want to start IMMEDIATELY!

LIFE AND DEATH FOODS

For your *Total Body Revolution* you need a Revelation to move from death to life, to move from the past to a glorious future. Never just "leave something behind" until you are ready to "pick up" or "start" something new. The **new** you should be nothing like the **old** you.

Leave behind alcohol and pick up smoothies and Kombucha. Leave behind fried chicken and pulled pork sandwiches and pick up black bean burgers, humus, stuffed avocados and sweet potato chips. Leave behind hamburgers, French fries and sodas and pick up a salad with all types of vegetables, fruit and nuts topped with Balsamic Vinegar and olive oil.

My wife and I do not go to fried chicken or seafood or bar-b-que restaurants; there is not much we want to eat there anymore. Our grocery cart is full of fresh vegetables and fruit, and very seldom if ever any meat, eggs, cheese or dairy. I recently attended a work party that featured bar-be-que beef sandwiches, baked beans, coleslaw and cookies; I was the only one in the building who did not eat the beef sandwich.

I am motivated to live a clean and healthy life. I want to live without being chained to a pillbox full of drugs. I desire to be disease free, living without pain. My life is worth forgoing death foods, so I may live a long, healthy life.

Have I eaten death foods in the past? Yes, I sure did! I have eaten way too much death foods for too many years; but that is in my past, a past to which I refuse to return. My journey from death to life has been a gradual one but intensifies and quickens as I research the consequences of eating death and the rewards of eating life. Leave your past in your past. To be a *Revolutionary,* change and become a new person.

LIFE AND DEATH "PEOPLE"

We do not abandon people, family, friends, co-workers or anyone else; we begin to naturally distance ourselves from them if they behave contrary to our beliefs and practices. Case in point, although you no longer drink alcohol, you can still hang out with your drinking friends and go to parties or restaurants that serve alcohol; yet by your not consuming any of these beverages you may not be invited back to these gatherings. Without "preaching" to them, you may be perceived as weird or fanatical for practicing your *Revolutionary* beliefs and thereby shunned by your peer group; but you are living an example of a changed life.

As you progress in your *10-Day Total Body Revolution* and continue past the 10-Days, you will seek out methods to stay the course and not fall back into your unhealthy lifestyles. You naturally migrate to people who have similar viewpoints, mannerisms and practices. It is normal NOT to go to bars and fast food restaurants because they do not serve what you desire.

Live your life before those who believe and act differently. Do not preach your new life-simply live it. Your life will speak for you. Be who you are, live your new life. Be infectious in your beliefs, attitude and new style. Actions speak louder than words.

LIFE AND DEATH "BELIEF SYSTEMS"

You are beginning to eat less often death foods. You associate less often with "death" people. In your *Revolution* you are *evolving* away from death "belief and practice systems". ANY system that is holding you back from you fulfilling your God given potential, your dreams, your vision or your passion is a death belief system.

Your mind must be renewed, changed and altered to think differently. Positive thinking and speaking comes from a healthy brain and strong body. Yes, there are many negative persons who are strong, but a truly *Revolutionized* person is drug free, does not criticize others, helps people to fulfill their greatest potential and sees the best in others.

"Life" belief systems will direct you away from hurtful, negative people and relations. "Life" belief systems draw you towards organizations and associations that seek to build people up, provide encouragement and cross cultural, racial and any type of demographic barrier.

Analyze your belief systems. Your new "life" belief systems cannot ostracize, belittle, divide or discriminate; you now bring life to everyone you encounter through every aspect of your existence. You are a new person both inside and out; you are revolutionized!

LIFE AND DEATH HABITS

Tradition, culture, family practices and habits are loved and cherished, but they cannot become a death habit.

Until a few years ago, I allowed my tradition and culture to dictate Thanksgiving would be a huge turkey and Christmas the same (amongst all the other events of the holidays). Most of the foods, prepared the way they were, I now view as death foods and I do not eat them. I no longer participate in these large family gatherings mainly because many of the family members are all dead due to their eating of death foods all their life.

If your family or culture dictates you eat and drink a certain way, do not discontinue the gatherings, but simply eat differently. Prior to attending any special get-togethers, eat a full meal of your food at home. Then when you attend the event eat extremely little of the presented death foods, if you cannot respectfully refrain from eating any of them. I always respect the host and hostess of events, yet I eat and drink as little as possible if I have to eat their food.

My life does not include many family or cultural gatherings; it does, however include meals and meetings with people who have death habits. I choose to eat, talk and act different than my associates because of my beliefs. I do not brow beat them to believe what I believe. When I am asked why I do not eat what they do or asked if a certain food is healthy, I explain my position in a short, concise, uplifting and positive manner. I influence them with my optimistic mannerisms and consistent actions.

Allow your actions to speak for themselves. You are noticed as a *Revolutionary* because of your practices. People will want to be a *Revolutionary* like you when they see the changes in your life.

<u>CONCLUSION</u>

I refuse to participate in death habits or rituals that have killed many people I have known and loved. I alter my life to new life habits, beliefs, people and foods that nourish my spirit, soul and body so I may be a living example of a *Revolutionary*.

The past truly stays in my past. I smile when I think of the family gatherings of my youth and I talk about the huge amount of foods I used to eat; but I do not desire to return to those days. I miss the family and friends who died because they did not change their lifestyle. I steel myself to not end up like them: sick, addicted to pills and shots and unable to live a long *Revolutionary* life.

Be a *Revolutionist*! Change all the "death" practices and beliefs to "life" practices and beliefs.

<u>Yes you can!</u>

CHAPTER 10

YOUR NEW MIND: BEING POSITIVE: YES YOU CAN

Having a positive attitude is of extreme importance. The glass is half full, not empty. You look for something good to happen, not expect something bad. We are happy when something good happens for someone and do not think "why did this not happen for me?" Your *Total Body Revolution* includes your attitude and being a positive, up person; yes you can!

A POSITIVE CONFESSION

The power of positive thinking, speaking and confession cannot be underestimated or understated. There are innumerable books available for your review by great scholars on the subject. Many models, formulas, routines and practices are espoused for your "inner healing" and revitalization.

My suggestions for everything are based upon common sense and practicability. Regardless of excuses and reasons why you cannot do something; I like to say, *"Dream Bigger and Do It"*! Alter your life. Alter your experiences. Go cold turkey if you must. Just do what you need to do. Become the new person you have always wanted to become.

Break free of the thought chains and belief structures that hold you bound. Anytime you begin to think negative, turn your thoughts and heart around to being positive. Think well of people, look for good not evil and make the time to be a friend to people in need.

Your positive confessions on life styles, food choices, mannerisms and behaviors will be contrary to most people you encounter. Most people are negative so your being positive will cause them to rethink their attitudes.

<u>A POSITIVE ATTITUDE</u>

Your positive confession with a positive attitude is a divergence of behavior for those in your "old" circle of relationships.

An attitude is a settled way of thinking or feeling about someone or something, typically one that is reflected in a person's behavior. Cultivate a new, positive way of thinking and speaking and then your new creative, passionate attitude will come forth in original abundant manifestations.

You are not a fake person, so do not pretend or put on a show.

If you are "in your right mind" you may be on the path of having a "renewed mind". This may be a sign that you are changing. Embrace change.

Be real. Learn how to perceive beauty amid ashes, how to alter your mind's eye. Revolutionizing your life will adjust the life path of those in your circle. This infectious and positive lifestyle will transform others more than you ever imagined.

This new attitude is attained or realized by accomplishing all the admonitions in this book and applying them to not only 10 days, but to the rest of your life. *A* 10-Day *Revolutionary* does not change the world, nonetheless a *10-Day* after *10-Day* after *10-Day* for-the-rest-of-your-life-Revolutionary, with an altered consciousness transforms everyone.

Revolution begins with this new attitude, which leads to a confession of a positive belief system. This metamorphosis redefines you and your environment preparing the way for a redefined life.

<u>A POSITIVE SELF-IMAGE</u>

When you become this new person others will want to emulate your transformation. You become infectious with hope, zeal and passion, bringing change to the "old" social order.

Your new life, your manifesto for change is crucial for society. As you take on the mantle of a transformed person you spread your characteristics to all peoples.

Through your changed thought processes, belief systems, eating and drinking habits, exercise routines and positive approach to all aspects of life you become a *Revolutionary*. This happens by believing in yourself and acting upon your beliefs.

You are not the "old" you, forever discard that belief system; you are a changed person-a renewed mind has brought a restored body and soul. The new you speak to large groups, opening their hearts, minds and souls to a new thought process and way of living that changes them into Revolutionaries.

Believe, see the difference, step out, overcome "normalcy" embody life, live revitalized and infect your community.

<u>CONCLUSION</u>

You are beautiful inside and out. Step out of your cocoon and become the person God intended you to be. Fear destroys the mind and stagnates life; this is your past not your present or future. You are a new "creature" a new "being" so walk out your newness with a fiery, communicable love.

CHAPTER 11

CONCLUSION: YOUR NEW DAILY SCHEDULE

Your new daily schedule is totally different than your old life. Your new mindset is totally different than your old mindset. Your new body is transforming itself daily into that which you have desired for all of your life.

You are being transformed into a radical, revolutionary person. In leaving your past behind you and adopting a positive belief system, you become available to transform the lives of everyone in your circle.

<u>**YOUR NEW DAILY SCHEDULE OF EATING AND DRINKING**</u>

Eating live food, not "death" foods keep you from ingesting trauma, toxins and drugs thereby keeping your soul and body clean. Decreasing to the elimination of ingesting meat, dairy and eggs will chart a course of health and stamina that heretofore you have never experienced.

Drinks full of life, energy, nutrition and purity cleanse and heal your body. Every day you drink plenty of water and get nourished with smoothies, herbal teas and Kombucha.

You are purging greasy fried foods, pastries, alcohol, tobacco, any type of sweet drinks and excess empty carbohydrates from your lifestyle. Now you fill your life with a wide variety of nuts, seeds, beans, peas, vegetables and fruit. Experimenting with new herbs and spices, learning how to sauté foods, how to use a crock-pot, how to broil and bake vegetables and acclimate your body to new types of foods and drinks sets you onto your revolutionary course of total body health.

Utilize the tools of fasting and herbal supplements. Research and experiment with the length of times you fast and the types of 100% organic herbal supplements, which are best for you.

<u>YOUR NEW DAILY SCHEDULE OF EXERCISE</u>

Begin each day stretching and develop a positive mentality to exercising. Throughout the day walk more and no matter what time of the day, you make time to work out! Aerobic, anaerobic and HITT are what you now do daily. During this *10-Day Total Body Revolution* you spend between thirty and forty-five minutes daily working out.

After the *10-Day Revolution*, as you continue with the program, take a break every 4th day from the fitness center for your body to recuperate; but do not stop exercising. If you are obese you need to exercise and radically change your lifestyle eating and drinking. Both aspects are necessary for your altered new existence.

<u>YOUR NEW DAILY SCHEDULE OF FORGIVENESS AND ACCOUNTABILITY</u>

The past is the past, learn from it, but do not relive it. Do not allow hurts, sorrow, rejection, and abuse or neglect to follow you into your future. Regardless of the outcome of past actions, move on. Get qualified counsel if needed.

Widen your circle of friendships and accountability partners. You must allow people whom you trust to speak into your life to help you develop into the person you need to become. Everyone at home, work, church, the grocery store, the restaurant and everywhere else you frequent is waiting on you to take your leadership *Revolutionary* place.

Forgive, let go and become accountable, as you do you become a *Revolutionary*.

YOUR NEW DAILY SCHEDULE OF TAKING BACK YOUR STOLEN LIFE

Taking back what was stole from you is accomplished by your attitude and actions. Forgiveness, accountability, declaring your freedom and being filled with love and purpose in life are all parts of your retrieving your life. This is achieved through a positive outlook on self and life and a determination to move forward.

Set you mind like flint, heart determined, and have life goals clearly established (write and post your goals where you see them daily); take back your life. Through your positive mannerisms, confession and actions all birthed in your reformed heart and mind, you change not only your life but also everyone around you.

Set in motion what is needed for change. Fight and take back what you need for the future, but leave behind anything that hinders. Consider your life and make the changes today for what you need to flourish and succeed.

THE FINAL CONCLUSION

Reread this book and read it over a third time. Go over a couple of times the chapters that introduced you to foreign concepts. Put as reminders all over your home, precepts from this book (speak positive, drink more water, the past is the past, be friendly, I am taking back what was stolen from me, etcetera).

Throw out toxic food and drink. Develop healthy relationships and expand your emotional support network.

Do not stop learning. Research your health condition (if any) and get medical tests run if you need then research alternative treatment options rather than settle for toxic and life-threatening pills, shots and/or surgical procedures. Ask questions, do not settle for negative prognosis; take charge of and change your life.

Be strong and steadfast in your new beliefs and practices. Do not allow your body to control what you eat, drink or do anymore. Do not allow your mind to say to you: be sarcastic, negative, complaining or alienate yourself from everyone. Do not allow your emotions to direct your responses to people who question your new practices. Be wise, informative, helpful and encouraging.

Begin now your *10-Day Total Body Revolution*, if you have not already. It may seem difficult, but if you want radical change you must act radically. If you must go slowly, go slowly; you have your whole life ahead of you to become whole.

As you begin your *Revolution*, know that you are not alone. There are many networks available that can help you in your *Revolution*.

Develop partnerships at work, church and your social groups-wherever you are to help others become *Revolutionaries*! Become infectious with your beliefs and practices and encourage others to step out and alter their lives. Be the instigator of change in your circle.

You are the agent of change, the *Revolutionary* that your ever-increasing circle of influence needs. You are becoming the leader you were born to be. Now live the life you want and need to live. Be the real you-the person of your dreams.

SELECTED BIBLIOGRAPHY

Suggested Readings

Holy Bible, New Living Translation, 2013, Carol Stream, Illinois, Tyndale House Publishers

Duke, James A, The Green Pharmacy, 1997, Emmaus, Pennsylvania, Rodale Press

Jakes, T. D., Lay Aside The Weight Taking Control of It Before It Takes Control of You! 1997, Tulsa, Albury Publishing.

Lerner, Ben, Body By God The Owner's Manual for Maximized Living, 2003, Nashville Tennessee, Thomas Nelson, Inc.

Levy, Thomas E., Curing the Incurable, 2002, Henderson Nevada, Livon Books

Levy, Thomas E., Optimal Nutrition for Optimal Health, 2001, New York, New York, Keats Publishing.

Loomis, James, Passionate Lover of God, 2018, Createspace.

Loomis, Janie, Spirit of the Forerunner: A Cry Goes Out, 2018, Createspace.

Okemiri, Nkem, 12 Seed Principles For People With Dreams, 2011, Abuja, Nigeria, Back To Life Publications

ABOUT THE AUTHOR

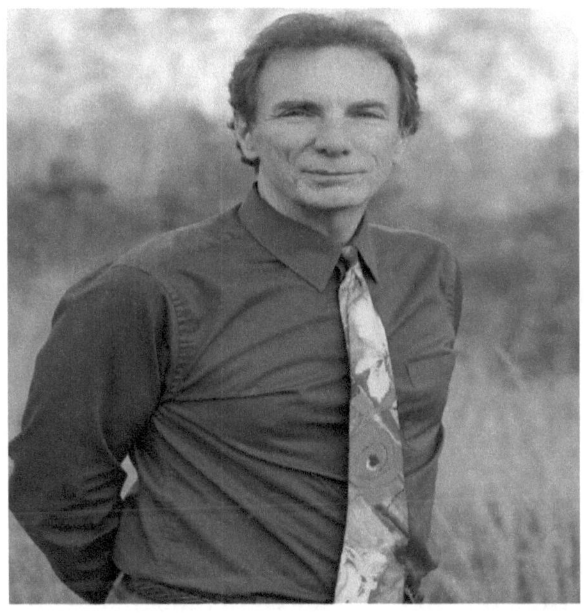

James Loomis is an auditor, a health and wellness columnist, nutritional researcher and a passionate lover of God. His health and wellness lectures are bold, hard hitting, fact and science based and convicting to all who want to hear the truth and learn how to become healthy and drug free. He and his wife Janie have been organic micro-farmers, gourmet foods manufacturers and marketers.

James and Janie are public speakers in secular and Christian seminars, are life-coaches, authors and fitness and health food fanatics.

James speaks with fire and conviction, humor and sensitivity on how to change one's circumstances and achieve personal success in every arena of life. He has seen countless people change their health through his instructions and lifestyle leadership in nutritional education.

He and Janie live in Atlanta, Texas.

Author photography by Elizabeth Howe of Fresh Wind Photography

Books by James and Janie Loomis are available via attending one of their conferences or seminars, on Amazon and through the website:
www.forerunnerspirit.com

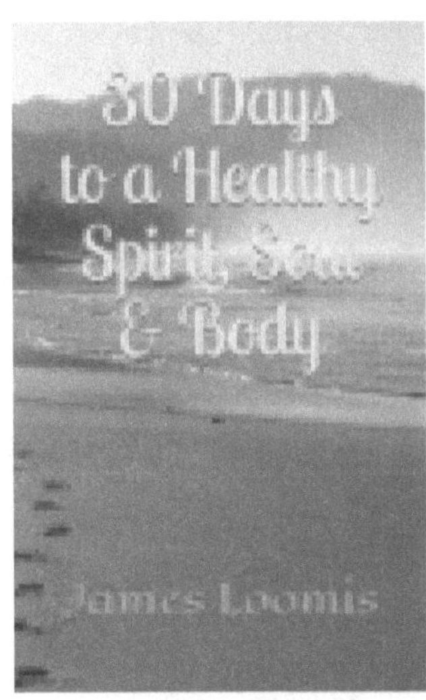

*<u>30 Days to a Healthy
Spirit, Soul & Body</u>*

- ❖ A daily devotional to strengthen your Spirit, Soul and Body.
- ❖ Healing of past wounds.
- ❖ Birthing hope in difficult situations.
- ❖ The motivational tool that sparks revival.
- ❖ The clarion call to a reinvigorated life.
- ❖ Awakening sleepers to their calling.
- ❖ Gentle, compelling and inspirational.
- ❖ Your tool for inner healing.
- ❖ Deliverance from soul-ties.

The carrier of God's Fire, Glory and Grace

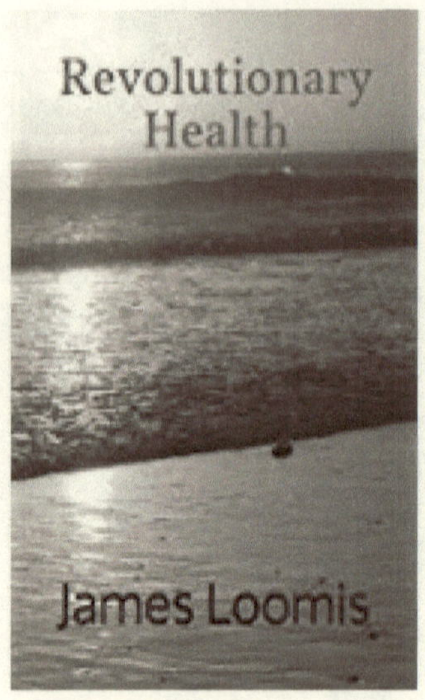

<u>**Revolutionary Health**</u>

❖   A 9-step plan for remission from cancer, heart disease and diabetes.

❖   A new way of thinking, speaking, eating and drinking.

❖   Your path to freedom from the bondage of obesity.

❖   A book of hope, encouragement and action on how to live drug free and healthy.

❖   Freedom from pain, illness and diets.

❖   A Radical/Revolutionary plan to prevent heart disease.

❖   Easy to follow with rewards of renewed strength, vitality and endurance.

❖   THE life you have always wanted.

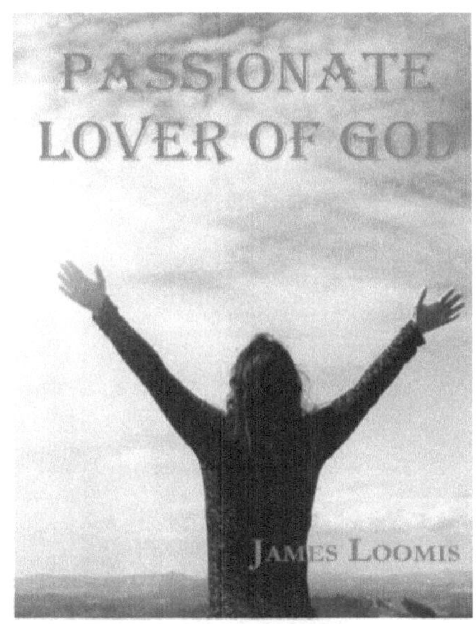

<u>PASSIONATE LOVER OF GOD</u>

--The tool you need to grow closer to God
--Your EVANGELISTIC tool to reach your world for Jesus
--The clarion call that awakens us to a deeper relationship with God
--The step-by-step guide you will want to share with everyone
--The clear point-by-point explanation on how to walk out your new intimate relationship with God
--Your mandate to draw intensely, passionately in love with Jesus
--The Bride of Christ cleansing herself for her soon wedding

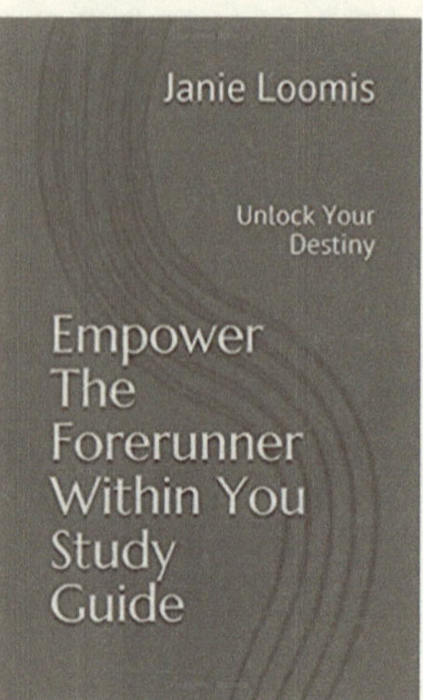

Empower the Forerunner Within You Study Guide

Are you a Forerunner? Has God chosen you to lead and direct His people? Are you stirred in your spirit to know more of the heart of God and bring His compassion to the world? Are you hungry to know more about activating this gift in your life? This book will empower and equip you. This Study Guide will open the door for your passage into the forerunner calling. Forerunners are hungry for God. They desire to propel people into their God given callings.

This book will awaken you; it will align you and help you to step into your position and authority as His Forerunner. Use this Study Guide in conjunction with the *Workbook and Journal* and you will be well prepared for the journey you have always dreamed of taking.

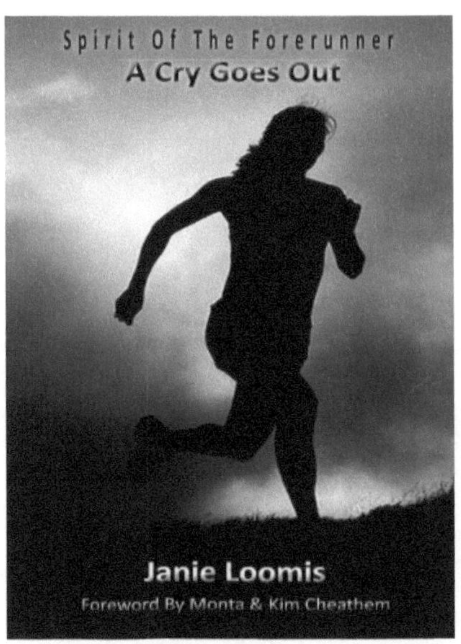

Spirit of the Forerunner: A Cry Goes Out

Intercession is a vital key to the prayer life of the Forerunner.
As Forerunners, we are to help the body of Christ understand their place on the world scene.
Forerunners are deeply prophetic and take very seriously the prophetic call on their lives.
As we draw closer to God in our worship, we begin to see as He sees, touch as He touches and know what He knows.
As we draw close to Him, we hear His heart.

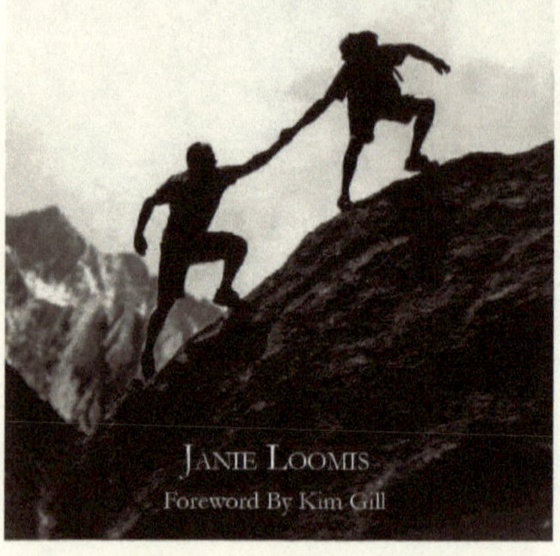

<u>Spirit of the Forerunner:</u>
<u>The Legacy of One Who Has Gone Before</u>

It is only through an obedient and humble spirit that God can use us for His glory.
If you are holding on to a word or promise from God, become obstinate, resolute and firm in belief that the promise is coming about and it is God's will to be done!
The key is our stepping out in faith. Have you taken a "leap of Faith"?
The Forerunner has been called and anointed by God to speak for the Father, use your voice, speak with the authority He has placed upon your calling.
People will see the anointing on your life and be drawn to it.

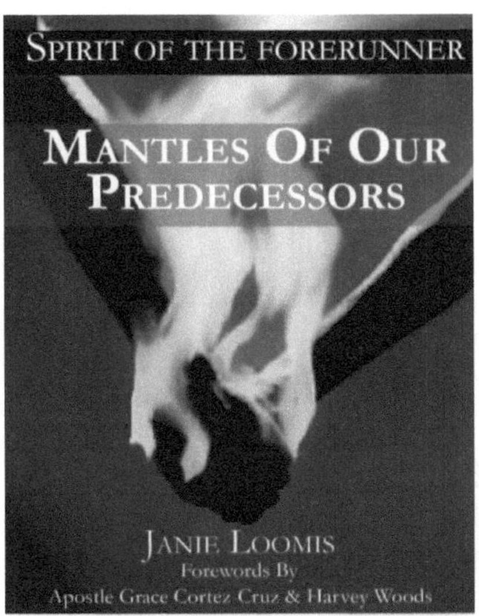

Spirit of the Forerunner: Mantles of our Predecessors

When you walk in the anointing of the forerunner, Holy Spirit causes the fire of God to consume people. Think beyond impossible and shake heaven and earth for the sake of your call.

Lock your eyes on the prize and look with spiritual understanding into your future.

This, the final book within the spirit of the Forerunner series, completes the calling and enables you to step out under the power and anointing given to the forerunner. As you walk cloaked with the mantle of our predecessors, you will gain confidence in your vocation and understand the importance of the forerunner in God's kindgom plan.